Identifying and Treating Mental and Emotional Disorders

Conditions of Neurosis and Psychosis

By: James M. Lowrance © 2010

TABLE OF CONTENTS:

Identifying and Treating Mental and Emotional Disorders

INTRODUCTION:

In the chapters that follow, I will present information regarding common emotional conditions of "neurosis" and the less-common conditions of mental illness referred-to as "psychosis". It is my intention to help define the differences between these two types of emotional and mental disorders but to also present the differences between common conditions of neurosis that are in the anxiety and depression categories.

Subjects covered include descriptions of major depression, bipolar depression, schizophrenia and different types of major anxiety disorders. Signs, symptoms and diagnosis are discussed, as well as the treatments that are administered for these different types of disorders (i.e. pharmaceutical, psychiatric and natural therapies).

It is my hope that this audiobook will provide a good basic educational resource for listeners wishing to learn about identifying and treating mental and emotional disorders.

CHAPTER ONE:

Psychosis versus Common Anxiety and Depression

Common anxiety and clinical depression are types of "neurosis". Psychosis is the term for a mental disorder that causes a person to lose touch with reality and that may cause them to have hallucinations and delusions. Mental disorders that are in the psychosis category include types of bipolar disorder and schizophrenia. Anxiety and common clinical depression are both in the neurosis category, meaning they are stress and nerve-related and not typically caused by a severe underlying mental disorder.

Persons with severe forms of depression, such as bipolar disorder, may have psychotic episodes but the more common type of clinical depression and anxiety disorders are not in the psychosis category, but rather are types of neurosis (psychoneurosis). According to the National Institute of Mental Health, psychosis affects an estimated 1% of the U.S. population, while the more common anxiety and depression conditions affect a much higher percentage. Perhaps as many as 1 in 4 or 25% of the American population experience an anxiety disorder and/or clinical depression at some time during their lives.

Anxiety-related "depersonalization" and "de-realization" can be mistaken for psychotic episodes. Depersonalization is an anxiety-induced experience in which a person feels he or she is "unreal" or no longer exists as a person (a sensation rather than a true delusion). They may even feel (but not actually believe) that they are no longer visible to other people and that others around them remain real but they no longer are.

Some anxiety patients describe it as feeling like they are watching their own actions from outside of themselves, and they no longer feel like a human being but have become robotic. Patients have described episodes, for example, of looking at their own face in a mirror and wondering if they are really there. They may also feel as if they no longer recognize themselves and feel as if they are having an identity crisis.

De-realization, is similar, except that the person's surroundings seem to lose reality. With de-realization, an anxiety sufferer will have episodes of experiencing feelings that their surroundings have become unreal. They may also feel as if reality itself is no longer something they can fully recognize during these moments (a feeling but not actually a belief). They may also question the reality of many things at these times, and may begin to wonder if life is simply a dream of some type. Some anxiety sufferers describe this experience as being like "living inside a bubble", or like they are trying to see everything through a haze or a thick fog. This is also referred to as "brain fog" when it hinders the ability for a person to concentrate with the same sharpness, as when they are not experiencing unreality symptoms.

Anxiety sufferers need to understand the fact that unreality symptoms do not indicate that they are going insane or actually losing touch with reality. They are sensations rather than actual manifestations of losing touch with reality in the true sense, as occurs with psychotic illnesses. They are both very common occurrences in anxiety sufferers, especially in those who experience panic attacks but will not cause damage to a person's mind or sanity. They are in fact a manifestation of the "fight or flight response" anxiety mechanism.

The fear of going insane is a very concerning one to people who experience severe anxiety and panic, and also to those who experience major/clinical depression. Indeed, anxiety and panic often co-exist, but these are irrational thoughts that will not happen.

Catastrophic Thinking

Mood disorder sufferers may experience episodes of "catastrophic thinking", but this symptom is also not related to true psychosis, although people with psychotic conditions can exhibit this manifestation. Catastrophic thinking happens to many anxiety sufferers and is also referred to as the "what ifs" (fear of possible events). Anxiety disorder patients describe thoughts of losing control of their selves in front of others and making their selves look silly or foolish. Other patients may experience a fear that they might pass out and need the aid of an ambulance, but that they will not be found in time by someone who can call one for them. Other anxiety sufferers have described fears of snapping and committing violence to other people around them, or that they might run down a grocery store isle, screaming or fall to the floor and curl up in a ball.

One of the reasons catastrophic thinking is so unpleasant is because these fearful thoughts can increase and intensify the already-present anxiety symptoms. Catastrophic thinking, in fact, can be a trigger for panic episodes in some people who struggle with it. This "what if" thinking tends to lead from one thought to another, until many fearful thoughts are all happening simultaneously, which could be referred to as a snowball type effect. The thoughts gain momentum and loom larger and scarier to the anxiety sufferer, as they increase during episodes of intense anxiety.

Identifying and Treating Mental and Emotional Disorders

To repeat, common anxiety and depression can have serious symptoms of their own, but they do not cause patients to become delusional or hallucinate in the true sense. This is the major difference between neurosis and psychosis.

Some bipolar cases are more severe than others and some patients are treated with only an antidepressant like an SSRI (Selective Serotonin Reuptake Inhibitor) while others may also need an anti-psychotic drug. With proper, ongoing treatment, bipolar patients can lead normal, productive lives.

CHAPTER TWO:

A Description of Schizophrenia and Bipolar Disorder

Schizophrenia is an illness affecting the mind and emotions that causes episodes of delusions, hallucinations and fragmented thinking or detached thoughts. This form of mental illness is treatable and treatments can actually reduce symptoms of psychosis to a degree that patients can live relatively normal lives. It is very important however, that treatment is adhered-to exactly as scheduled because missed doses of drug therapies can hinder the effects of them.

There are certain diseases that can be mistaken for schizophrenia, including thyroid disorders, especially the ones called "Hashimoto's Encephalopathy" (an acute neurological disease) and "Thyroid Storm". The same is true of severe nutritional deficiencies that can cause psychosis until diagnosed and treated. Severe Vitamin D deficiency for example has been identified as a cause of schizophrenia in medical research studies and correction of it via Vitamin D replacement therapy can resolve it.

In these type cases, treating underlying medical disorders can cure the mental illness but when schizophrenia does not have an underlying cause but is "idiopathic" (its own disorder - no secondary cause), it is lifelong and requires ongoing treatment.

A Description of Bipolar Disorder

The major features of bipolar disorder are different from common clinical depression. The name "bipolar disorder" describes "two opposite extremes".

People with this mental disorder will have episodes of severe depressed mood, followed by episodes of manic behavior (mania, meaning periods of extreme, elated feelings). In fact during manic episodes, a bipolar person may seem full of energy and want to go on late-night shopping sprees for example, or work on a new project for long hours. They may also go without sleep for many days or even weeks at a time. Bipolar depressive disorder was previously referred to as "manic depression" because of the episodes of mania that are a characteristic feature of it.

Bipolar disorder patients tend to feel self-exalted at these manic times, thinking they are very special and greater/stronger than the average person, which is a type of delusional thinking. Some bipolar people have "mixed episodes", in which these severely depressed and manic spells may cycle more rapidly, rather than occurring weeks apart.

Can Bipolar Disorder be Misdiagnosed?

If you have extremely depressed episodes, followed by extremely elated episodes (manic/mania), this can point strongly toward bipolar disorder. If you instead have anxiety symptoms that alternate with depression, this would not be bipolar because anxiety is a fear or worry emotion and not one of elation/mania. So, if you cycle between great sadness and an exaggerated happiness that is not triggered by events going on in your life, you may indeed have bipolar disorder.

Some people who exhibit episodes of extreme depression, with alternating episodes of anxiety that causes others around them to misperceive their nervous energy as "mania" may cause them to believe they are experiencing bipolar, when they are not.

Identifying and Treating Mental and Emotional Disorders

Doctors who do not specialize in mental health, have been known to misdiagnose sufferers of combined anxiety and depression, due this very type of mistaken observation.

There are some theories that suggest drug and/or alcohol abuse can actually cause bipolar disorder in susceptible people over time. It is otherwise believed to be a brain abnormality that one is born-with but that may not manifest until young adulthood. When I say "born with" this can actually mean that the abnormal components in the brain are present at birth but it might not be developed enough to cause the characteristic mood swings until early childhood, adolescence or in the early adult years.

How Do You Support a Person with Bipolar Disorder?

Bipolar patients need total support that they can sense and feel from you by being available to listen when they need to talk and offering words of encouragement to them as often as necessary. Also giving them space to be alone when they legitimately need private time to themselves and when there is no danger that they will harm their self. Reassuring them that their drug therapy is essential to their ongoing health and that it is helping them to retain a better quality-of-life is also important.

Complimenting them, on their accomplishments and encouraging them to continue achieving personal goals as they are able to do so is also part of this. Reminding them that they are not "insane" or "crazy" but that they have a mental illness which does not take away from their inward character or intelligence can be beneficial as well.

Letting them know often that you love them if your relationship allows, is also important.

Bipolar is possibly something one has at birth as previously mentioned and is a lifelong disorder when idiopathic. Some medical research has shown that the brains of bipolar patients reveal differences from that of the healthy general public but no definitive conclusions have been made as yet in regard to these brain differences. Despite it being a lifelong disorder, it may not manifest in some people until adult years. Most cases will become evident by the time a person reaches their early twenties, according to mental health research experts.

What are the Differences between Bipolar Disorder Types I and II?

Both conditions present with severe episodes of depression, also referred-to as clinical or major depression and both also present with the opposite pole of emotion, being that of "mania", which are episodes of elation that alternate with the depression. Bipolar II is differentiated due to its less pronounced manic episodes. They refer to these less severe mania symptoms as "hypomania" because it falls short of causing the severity of mania that those with "bipolar I" have. People with "bipolar II" are also less-prone to experience delusions and/or hallucinations (psychotic episodes).

To repeat, bipolar in-general would not simply be depressed mood but would be severely depressed mood, alternating with episodes of an exaggerated mood of elation.

Bipolar patients have very unstable moods that go very low and then very high and during the high or "manic" episodes, they may feel greater and mightier than others around them (delusional beliefs). The depressed moods can be so severe, as to land a bipolar person in bed for days or weeks at a time and the manic episodes can keep them from sleeping for periods that long as well. The goal of treatment is to get the moods on a more even level so that the peaks and valleys are no longer occurring.

CHAPTER THREE:

Confirming a Diagnosis of Mental Illness

Recently, while I was moderating on a thyroid disease, patient-forum, someone posted about being diagnosed by an MD, with "Bipolar Disorder" and they were prescribed an anti-psychotic drug for this. While these type drugs are extremely needful and very helpful to people who do truly need them for disorders of psychosis they may be suffering, at the same time, I believe any patient in doubt about a diagnosis of this type, should seek confirmation of needing such a drug. Sometimes a second opinion by a qualified mental health professional is needed because these drugs are powerful and designed for a specific purpose and should only be prescribed to patients who actually have psychotic disorders or episodes.

Below is my response to this individual, in regard to Bipolar Disorder and in regard their being prescribed drugs for this, despite their concerns that the diagnosis could possibly be incorrect. Some of my response to this, came from my own experience in seeing family members diagnosed with psychotic disorders they did not have and from an experience years ago, when this was also my personal experience. Following below, is the reply I gave this person who posted on that forum:

My Reply:

"While I certainly believe these type drugs can be of tremendous value to people who have Bi-Polar Disorder or schizophrenia, I also know that for reasons we may never know, there are Doctors who are prescribing some of these anti-psychotic drugs to people who do not have the disorders the drugs are designed to treat.

Identifying and Treating Mental and Emotional Disorders

I believe the prescription drug "Depakote" that your Doctor is prescribing for you, is also used to treat epilepsy and migraine headaches.

I know a little about the phenomenon of non-confirmed diagnosis of mental disorders because I have a nephew and aunt on opposite sides of my family, who were both "diagnosed" with bi-polar and schizophrenia and neither of them had either of these disorders. Their incorrect diagnoses were corrected once they were evaluated further by qualified mental health professionals.

In regard to my personal experience in this area, in the late 1980s, I had a very bad job situation and developed anxiety and a stomach malady due to the stress of it and upon seeing an MD, he diagnosed me with manic depression (an early term for bi-polar disorder). He prescribed me an anti-psychotic drug, which I only took for one month, until my Church Pastor, made me realize it was a bogus diagnosis and he proved this by showing me a medical resource describing the condition in-detail. I experienced severe side effects from the drug as well, during my short term use of it. My symptoms did not even remotely point to bi-polar but were typical anxiety symptoms, which resolved after a job change, to a less stressful occupation.

Let me just say that with bi-polar, the name describes just what it is, "two opposed extremes". People with it, will become severely depressed, and followed by episodes of "mania" as previously described. The point being, that if you do not experience spells of mania/extreme elation, it is unlikely Bi-polar Disorder. Another reason I know this is because I have witnessed the episodes experienced by people who are bi-polar and it is fairly obvious when a person actually has this mental disorder.

Identifying and Treating Mental and Emotional Disorders

Depression alternating with anxiety is not the same thing. These two commonly co-exist but anxiety is not mania, it is a fear emotion, that also causes chronic worry at times and certainly this would not be an elated or exalting feeling.

In regard to schizophrenia, this mental disorder is characterized by episodes of hallucinations, delusional thinking and losing touch with reality. Patients with this condition can many times have their psychosis well controlled through anti-psychotic medications and they can live relatively normal lives. This does vary however among patients, according to the severity of their disorders. In more severe cases patients may be required to receive ongoing professional care in a mental health facility.

Neither bipolar nor schizophrenic patients are "crazy" or "insane". These are unfair and inconsiderate characterizations of them. These patients are experiencing mental illnesses, of no fault of their own and can be as high quality in their character and as intelligent as anyone who does not suffer mental illness.

I would be very cautious when doubting a suspect-diagnosis to add such a drug (anti-psychotic prescription) to your treatment regimen and for a more definitive, substantiated diagnosis I would see a mental health professional before accepting one offered by an MD or GP who does not specialize in mental health. Anxiety and depression affect a very large percent of the population, while bi-polar and schizophrenia affect approximately 1%.

ALSO: yes, depression and anxiety both are strongly connected and are common symptoms of thyroid disease as you asked in your question. Bi-polar is believed to have a connection to thyroid disease as well but as I describe above, it must meet the mania criteria to be diagnosed bi-polar disorder.

Identifying and Treating Mental and Emotional Disorders

Depakote, in my understanding is designed to control the mania aspect of the disorder.

Regular MDs and GPs, in my opinion, should be cautious in diagnosing common anxiety and depression, as psychotic disorders."

(End of Reply)

How Do Sufferers of Bipolar Depression Appear Emotionally?

A bipolar person will look profoundly sad at times and as if they are unable to enjoy their self. They may also look very tired and lacking in energy and will often avoid being around other people. This is a description of their depressed phase.

In their mania phase, they will appear very elated and happy, to an exaggerated extent and seem to have an endless supply of energy at these times. They may also seem very creative at these times and want to work on projects endlessly or go on shopping sprees. They may also seem to be unable to relax and may avoid sleeping for days or even weeks at a time.

In-short, a bipolar person will appear extremely depressed, followed by episodes of appearing to be exaggeratedly happy. It is a condition affecting the emotions and has to do with extreme sadness, followed by exaggerated feelings of elation and happiness.

17

A personality disorder on the other hand, has to do with how one relates to other people, their treatment of them, and their reactions to them, how they show affection toward them and whether or not they exercise manipulation type behaviors toward others. Some people have both emotional disorders and personality disorders at the same time.

CHAPTER FOUR:

Cognitive Behavioral Therapy (CBT) for Anxiety Disorders

Anxiety Disorders include Panic Disorder, Obsessive-Compulsive Disorder, Post-Traumatic Stress Disorder, Generalized Anxiety Disorder, and Phobias (social phobia, agoraphobia, and specific phobia). Approximately 40 million American adults ages 18 and older, or about 18.1 percent of people in this age group in a given year, have an anxiety disorder. Anxiety disorders frequently co-occur with depressive disorders or substance abuse. Most people with one anxiety disorder also have another anxiety disorder. Nearly three-quarters of those with an anxiety disorder will have their first episode by age 21. (Statistics are from the U.S. NIMH)

As terrible as anxiety feels, it is neither harmful nor dangerous. Using that sentence as a search, you'll see multiple sites confirming this and learning this fact is an aspect of CBT. Anxiety is a natural emotion, created to help us flee from danger or to perform more powerfully for an important task (fight or flight response). With "anxiety disorder" this mechanism happens at the wrong times (out of context), like at the grocery store check out stand, in crown of people etc... Anxiety and depression commonly co-exist; in fact more people with anxiety disorders have a degree of depression than don't. Anxiety will not make you go crazy; no matter how often you experience it and will not cause physical damage, unless you already have serious underlying health problems. It heightens bodily functions the same as exercise does. Anxiety is not stress; it is a manifestation of stress and is the body's way of trying to shed-off stressful things by allowing the body to react to them.

Sometimes with strong anxiety emotions, people experience "depersonalization and/or derealization", in which you feel unreal or everything around you feels unreal (unreality symptoms) as previously mentioned. This is not a sign of insanity; it is common with anxiety and depression. Anxiety will not progress to schizophrenia or insanity because it is "neurosis" and not "psychosis" which are two completely different things. People with "psychosis" may have no anxiety or depression at all.

Psychosis is defined by delusions and hallucinations. Anxiety suffers can have mild hallucination-type experiences but is the minds way of trying to locate a perceived danger and is still not the same as true psychosis. These facts comforted me greatly at times of severe anxiety I experienced with the onset of Hashimoto's thyroiditis (autoimmune thyroid disease) that first manifested with severe anxiety and panic symptoms.

Cognitive Behavioral Therapy is one of the more successful treatments for anxiety symptoms. Many anxiety disorder patients have had great success in overcoming and coping with anxiety symptoms through this method.

Aspects of CBT that are important parts of the therapy include the three following:

CBT helps change the way one thinks about anxiety in general and about the symptoms it causes. The patient will learn through this aspect of CBT that anxiety itself is a "natural emotion". The unpleasantness of the symptoms in people in whom anxiety has become a "disorder" comes from the fact that this normal emotion can occur out of context or at inappropriate times (disordered).

When a patient learns that the emotion he is experiencing is not "strange or foreign," this alone can help toward reducing the fear of the symptoms anxiety disorder causes. Once a patient with anxiety accepts the fact the emotion is natural and is supposed to occur at the appropriate times, he can also work on other steps toward coping.

CBT looks at those things that have become "triggers" in causing anxiety to occur out of context or in a disordered fashion. One way to express this fact to an anxiety sufferer is to say: "Anxiety is a completely natural and normal emotion and it is only the timing of it that has become out of the order it was intended to happen." Under normal circumstances, the anxiety emotion was created to be triggered in order to allow the one experiencing it to have the sudden added strength and presence of mind, to flee from danger or to fight an enemy that has attacked him. This is the origin of the term for triggered-anxiety that is referred to as the "fight or flight" response.

Some anxiety research groups believe that social phobia for example, often begins in childhood and progresses as a person enters adulthood. The sympathetic nervous system response called (fight or flight response) begins to trigger inappropriately. Like other anxiety disorders, the negative responses a person has when feeling anxious about a social events or settings they are attending or planning to attend (immediate or anticipated anxiety), becomes more of a learned behavior. A person with Social Anxiety Disorder (SAD) for example, may experience panic attacks when socializing with one or more people or may avoid social settings because of their uncomfortable anxiety symptoms when around people. These reactions cause the anxiety disorder to worsen and it may eventually need drug and/or psychiatric therapy, for coping with it, or to possibly overcome it over time.

Identifying and Treating Mental and Emotional Disorders

People with SAD, develop fears of being judged by others whom they believe to be observing them closely, as to how well they converse with others and as to how well they display their social mannerisms. In reality, others are not observing them as closely as they think and are more comfortable around them than they believe they are. It is a type of extreme or exaggerated shyness that can seriously affect quality of life and the ability to cope in society. Sad can restrict a person's life so that they do not want to go out into public for any reason, including things like shopping for food or going to the post office, to a doctor visit, etc...

Entertainer - Donny Osmond is one famous sufferer of social phobia, with associated panic attacks that he attests to being present beginning in his childhood. He has however, learned to cope with SAD, through drug therapy and Cognitive Behavioral Therapy and has since served as a spokesman for people with anxiety disorders.

Recognize that anxiety also gives added abilities, determination and ambition to the one who experiences it, to perform tasks at hand. This can be any task that requires what some might also call "intestinal fortitude" - that internal strength we all have and must call upon at times, as it is needed. Everyone has important tasks to perform in their everyday lives and at times we also experience emergency situations or those with important priorities involved. Firemen must be on alert to put out fires that are called in to them, teachers must have the inspiration to interest their pupils in learning the subjects being studied, and an athlete in a track meet must be ready to run in an attempt to win a race. Without the anxiety emotion, they would not have the added strength and inspiration to accomplish these tasks as successfully.

A person who is called upon to make a public speech for example, needs that extra inspiration to bring forth his spoken points more powerfully and with conviction. Anxiety is what adds to this experience and helps them to accomplish this. The butterflies in the stomach and sweaty hands can actually be a sign that you one is about to make a powerful presentation and not that they are about to run off of the stage due to stage-fright and so, it is all in how one looks at it. You can make anxiety responses work for you or work against you. Will you see it as positive energy to help inspire you or as fear that is holding you back? That is the question. Herein lies the secret to this aspect of Cognitive Behavioral Therapy; the way in which one perceives the anxiety they are experiencing!

CHAPTER FIVE:

Positive Versus Negative Responses to Anxiety

When a group of people ride on a roller coaster at the amusement park, some will experience anxiety as an extreme fear-emotion while others on the same ride will experience it as welcome excitement. The types of people, who enjoy the adrenaline rush, also experience some fear with their excitement, but they actually enjoy it! They actually enjoy being scared occasionally and are the types of people who also like to take in a suspense thriller movie or horror film to get that same type of thrill. They are exhilarated by these experiences and one term used to describe them is "adrenaline junkies." If anxiety sufferers can learn to view anxiety in a different light and recognize it as a natural emotion, they can then use it to their advantage.

Getting anxiety to work more for you and less against you.

Is this more easily-said-than-done for people whose anxiety has developed into a disorder? Of course it is, but anything worthwhile takes time and effort to accomplish. An anxiety disorder sufferer who works on this important aspect will see small gains that will encourage him to continue in changing his perceptions about anxiety and over time, will begin to see a cumulative improvement in many areas of life that were previously affected negatively by anxiety.

An online search using "Cognitive Behavioral Therapy" as the search-term will yield lots of quality, reputable CBT programs that are available. Most are very affordable and well worth the cost for those seeking coping skills for anxiety disorders.

Unusual but Effective Methods for Coping with Panic Attacks

One method that some former panic attack sufferers have used is to not resist them but to actually invite them to occur. While this sounds strange at first glance, it is a method that in-essence tricks the "fight or flight" response into reversing itself. This anxiety mechanism thrives of resistance and fear; in fact these are triggers for panic attacks. By literally challenging anxiety to takes its best shot, you cause it to shut down because the fuel is not there for anxiety to run on.

Part of this method can also involve learning to flow with anxiety, so that you work with it, rather than it working against you. By practicing this aspect, one can eventually learn to channel anxiety into a positive direction, such as toward a creative process (i.e. art, sports, writing, etc...).

One PhD psychiatrist in the UK discovered that by having her patients to conjure up torrid romantic fantasies, they could stop anxiety and panic attacks in their tracks. Again, this is an unusual method but one that her patients found relief from anxiety by practicing. This would be more-so in the "Diversion Method" category and one that other psychiatrists have found effective in different versions for many years.

"Exposure therapy" is a method in which an anxiety sufferer exposes their self to those things that trigger their phobias. They do so gradually until the fear comes under their control and that will sometimes completely subside for them over time.

These methods take time and effort but can be effective in overcoming anxiety and panic attacks. It can also help to join anxiety forums and read & share personal anxiety experiences and coping-gains with fellow sufferers.

CHAPTER SIX:

What are the Differences between OCD and Generalized Anxiety Disorder? And What is Cyberchondria?

With Obsessive Compulsive Disorder, there is usually an "acting out" aspect in which you repeat certain rituals having to do with daily tasks such as washing your hands, turning off light switches, etc... These type things are very strong impulses with OCD sufferers because they feel they are not completing them thoroughly or completely enough. They may also obsess about something like germs getting on them and causing them illness and this will result in compulsive avoidance behaviors, such as not wanting to touch other people and not wanting to go outside of their homes without gloves or something covering their mouth and nose to prevent contracting germs.

When repeated thoughts that one obsesses about, remain the thought-real, without the acting-out aspect, this would likely be more-so in the "Generalized Anxiety Disorder" category in which chronic thoughts of worry is a key manifestation. With GAD, people do worry and obsess about things like illness, school, work, relationships and yes, some GAD sufferers report struggling with their firmly held beliefs. This is not a psychosis but rather is in the "neurosis" category, so is not actually a mental illness but rather a condition of chronic anxiety (thoughts of fear and worry).

By doing an online search using OCD and GAD as search terms and comparing the descriptions of the two and one will find that compulsive worry and racing thoughts are more-so in the GAD category, due to lack of the acting-out aspect that occurs with OCD.

Identifying and Treating Mental and Emotional Disorders

Cognitive Behavioral Therapy programs are available online via online search as well and patients can find coping though this type of therapy.

Is Cyberchondria a Real Anxiety Disorder?

The anxiety mechanism called "the fight or flight response", is an aspect of the "sympathetic nervous system" that is activated at inappropriate times, which is where the term "anxiety disorder" is derived from.

Those who through online search have come across worse-case scenarios for their physical symptoms, whether it occurs on a forum or even on the most reputable medical information websites can develop cyberchondria. I believe with conviction that warning should be given on medical information search sites in regard to researching medical and health information responsibly and in-balance. This type disclaimer needs added from time-to-time as a reminder on online patient-support resources as well, including forums and message boards. The fact that excellent support and information forums and medical information sites do exist is wonderful. I personally love them and have resorted to them many times for information regarding my own health disorders and to compile information for resources I have written.

If you do a search on "cyberchondria" (films on the subject are available on YouTube), it will give you a better sense of how serious the phobia from imbalanced information from online symptom-searches can be. To give an example; I read a thread posted by a man who was experiencing muscle twitching in one leg but reported no muscle weakness or atrophy.

The response he received was to the effect "That is concerning for ALS". The motor neuron disease called ALS (Amyotrophic Lateral Sclerosis) is a 100% fatal disease and most patients succumb to it within 2 to 3 years, with only a few going as long as 10 or longer (rare). Can you imagine the potential anguish that type of information might place on such an individual?

I'm a "patient advocate" and I have corresponded with 1,000s of patients since 2004 and I'm an author of many medical titles. I learned about trends over the years and one that has proven to be detrimental to the emotional health of some patients who conduct online searches regarding their symptoms, has been the cyberchonria issue.

Despite this, I am 100% for self-education in-balance and support forums and I always will be but I do believe there should be an ongoing awareness (reminders) of the possibility that some patients may be at risk for developing cyberchondria and we who post online certainly do not want to contribute to this very real anxiety disorder.

Microsoft conducted a study regarding cyberchondria, led by a computer scientist with a medical degree; here is a quote by him that is also found on the New York Times site:

"People tend to look at just the first couple results," Mr. Horvitz said. "If they find 'brain tumor' or 'A.L.S.,' that's their launching point."

It may seem at a first glance of this phenomenon that this is a rare happening but it is affecting an estimated "5%" of the population, which is huge. This is why occasional reference/warning to it should be given in regard to the potential for medical searches to contribute to chronic anxiety, in my opinion. Instruction on how to search reputable sources and comparing information for balance should also be a part of that.

CHAPTER SEVEN:

The Basic Differences between Anxiety & Depression

Anxiety and depression have a lot of similarities and some are even of the opinion that these are the same type fear-emotions that simply manifest differently in different people.

When you look at a list of symptoms for each there are indeed a great deal of similarities between them. Both can manifest with the following in-common symptoms.

- feelings of hopelessness
- agitation
- feeling withdrawn
- fatigue
- lack of ambition
- inability to enjoy things that used to bring pleasure
- fear of the future
- inability to cope with stressful situations

It is also true that anxiety and depression often co-exist, in fact persons with actual anxiety disorders almost always have a degree of depression, along with it and persons with clinical depression commonly have a degree of co-existing anxiety.

So what would be considered some major distinguishing features of each? The fact is, that many times they are not easily distinguishable, in fact many Doctors, such as MDs that are not also psychiatrists or psychologists (mental health specialists), many times find it difficult to distinguish between them.

So many times they will diagnose a patient with common emotional manifestations, as described above, as being a combination of both anxiety and depression or a "mixed emotional disorder".

One Anxiety Disorder that is more-so a mix of both anxiety and depression, than the others that exist, is "Generalized Anxiety Disorder". With this type anxiety, patients commonly experience a mix of both anxiety and depression. They may at times have stronger manifestations of depression and at other times, stronger manifestations of anxiety, while yet at other times, they are both about even in manifestation.

So what would be a major distinguishing feature of each that helps us to recognize the difference between the two? A major distinguishing feature of depression that is often listed as one of its major symptoms is "profound sadness". An anxiety sufferer sometimes experiences spells of emotion, that causes them to have crying spells etc.., but it is not the same profound sadness that is more chronically severe with depression. Anxiety sufferers on the other hand, have as a major feature of it, the "fear emotion", which can be the bewildering type, such as severe anxiety attacks or panic attacks or can be the chronic lingering type that manifests as chronic worry or severe apprehension.

The chronic worry aspect of anxiety, is what is most often mistakenly referred to as depression, when it is actually a fear emotion; fear of the future, fear about health, finances etc…, and though it is not in the depression category, it can result in depression, due to the prolonged periods of stress it causes.

To better illustrate this, let's look at a couple of example scenarios:

In the first example scenario, we have a man, with a very important business meeting coming up. In this meeting, he will be required to convince the heads of his company, that his past accomplishments merit him a promotion to a more important position with the firm.

The meeting is scheduled for two weeks away and yet the man has such hopes in doing well at the meeting, that he worries himself sick, during the entire two weeks leading up to the meeting. Family or friends observing his period of chronic worry, might make the observation, saying; "He sure has been depressed these past two weeks." The fact is that the man was experiencing a manifestation of anxiety, called chronic or obsessive worry, being triggered by a fear of failure.

In a second example scenario, we have a woman who does lose a long held position she had with a prestigious firm. This causes her to sink into a deep feeling of profound loss, that she feels she cannot recuperate from emotionally. She has continual feelings of sadness and has constant crying spells. An observer of her situation and resulting emotional state, remarks; "She has just been a bundle of nerves since losing her job and she's really going through an anxious time right now." In reality, the woman's experience is more-so in the depression category because she is experiencing profound sadness over losing her long held position with the firm.

While we may be able to better-place these examples of emotional scenarios into either the anxiety or depression categories, we also realize that both of these people very likely experienced aspects of both emotions to some degree.

Again, this demonstrates how closely related these emotions are and how they often co-exist and how they can also fuel each other, causing worsening symptoms of each.

Fortunately, there are treatments that can help to diminish the symptoms of both emotional disorders simultaneously, such as SSRI Antidepressants, designed to help patients who experience both anxiety and depression, or either of them. There are also treatments, such as "Cognitive Behavioral Therapy", that offers coping and overcoming skills, for both anxiety and depression.

CHAPTER EIGHT:

Antidepressants Effective for some but not for Others

Before I begin the next headings in regard to SSRI antidepressants and other psychotropic drugs, I feel it is important that I make it very clear that I believe in the effectiveness of these type drugs for the right patients and in the proper cases. I in-fact have close relatives who take these type prescribed drugs for anxiety disorders and major depression and they benefit significantly from them. Some patients in less common cases cannot adjust properly to certain types of these drugs however and must be given trials of different kinds to find the one that is appropriate for them.

The following are types of psychotropic drugs (anti-anxiety and antidepressant) that are commonly prescribed to help patients with mood disorder symptoms.

- Paxil
- Prozac
- Zoloft
- Wellbutrin
- Effexor
- Klonopin
- Ativan
- BuSpar
- Valium
- Xanax

If the drug you're taking, is not working as it should, as prescribed for anxiety, depression or mixed emotional disorder or it is causing unwanted side effects, you may need to discuss with your Doctor, slowly weaning off of the drug.

Considering a trial of an "as-needed" anti-anxiety medication, may hold the solution. These can be taken short-term, rather than the type that must be built-up in your system and maintained as a daily, permanent regimen. The fact is that some patients do fine with long-term antidepressants, while others do not.

Some Doctors seem to believe SSRI drugs (selective serotonin reuptake inhibitors) and other types of antidepressants work well for everyone but this simply is not true. I have corresponded with dozens of thyroid patients since the year 2003, who simply could not adjust well to them even after several months of trying to benefit from them, while many others report doing very well on them. People are individuals and nothing works exactly the same for everyone and is a common sense approach that both Doctors and patients should take with these type drugs.

Medication for bipolar disorder, which may include one or more of the drugs listed above, helps to level-out these two opposite poles so that the person doesn't experience the extreme peaks and valleys but is on a more even plane with their emotions. The poles in-essence come closer together rather than being so far apart.

When a bipolar patients stops taking their medication, these poles begin to spread apart again, so that extreme opposites in emotion are experienced, as occurred to them before treatment. This will result in times of withdrawal from others, profound sadness, lack of energy and need to sleep excessively and inability to enjoy things that once brought pleasure (major, severe depression). This will be followed by times of the person feeling highly energetic, erratic behavior, inability to sleep and working on projects endlessly (manic episodes).

Identifying and Treating Mental and Emotional Disorders

It is very important for bipolar patients not to stop their drug therapies because they can actually experience a worsening of these extremes of emotion when the leveling effect of the medication is suddenly halted. This is why some patients with bipolar and other mood disorders who stop their drugs cold turkey, display bizarre behaviors or develop suicidal or violent tendencies.

Can Anxiety and Depression Require Medical Treatments?

There are a number of medical causes for anxiety and depression including neurotransmitter imbalances (usually treated with SSRI drugs listed previously) and a qualified medical doctor can evaluate patients for these. Some of these causes would also include sex hormone imbalances, thyroid disorders, blood glucose imbalances and a common heart murmur called "Mitral Valve Prolapse" (often involves a nervous system imbalance called "dysautonomia").

While psychotropic drugs like antidepressants and anti-anxiety medications can be effective in treating mood disorders, if there is an underlying medical condition contributing-to or directly causing anxiety and/or depression symptoms, diagnosing and treating it can go further than any other treatment in resolving it.

If other causes are ruled-out, one can discuss with their doctor, a trial of a medication directed a relieving anxiety symptoms or psychiatric and self-help therapies that can help to accomplish this. Many anxiety patients benefit from a combination of both and in some cases can wean-off slowly from medication, once other therapies have gained them ample coping skills.

Identifying and Treating Mental and Emotional Disorders

SSRI antidepressants (drugs that regulate neurotransmitters in the brain) for example do not benefit everyone who is give a trial of them and some are switched to other types, such as non-addictive anti-anxiety medications, one called BuSpar (or generic-Busperone) being in that category.

Blood Testing Before Prescribing Antidepressants

I was one of those patients who, was suspected of having emotional problems, not being caused by an underlying medical problem. I ended up requesting my own blood tests because I suspected a medical problem or disease, even expressing this to the first Doctor I went to with my symptom complaints.

The combination of antidepressant, anti-anxiety medication and beta-blocker, that the first Doctor prescribed me in spite of my suggestion that I did not have an emotional-only disorder, did not help me. My symptoms actually became worse until my underlying thyroid disease was diagnosed and treated. Doctors are human and capable of mistakes like everyone else but it is situations like these that point to the need for more education by the general public on the importance of diagnostic testing for underlying medical conditions.

Many times anxiety and/or depression does not have a medical cause but if a patient has other physical symptoms that indicate a possible co morbid disease, they should have blood testing ordered to determine if a medical condition is the cause, or to rule it out. Treating symptoms alone, without treating an underlying medical condition that is causing them, will only do so much good or possibly none all. In a worse case scenario, medications for anxiety and depression alone, while leaving an underlying disease untreated may actually cause the patient's condition to become worse.

Identifying and Treating Mental and Emotional Disorders

CHAPTER NINE

Can Hypoglycemia and other Medical Conditions Mimic Psychiatric Disorders?

Glucose (blood sugar) is regulated in the body through the pancreas (endocrine gland that produces insulin) via the involuntary nervous system. While hypoglycemia (a sudden drop in blood glucose levels) doesn't mimic bipolar to a large degree, a person can experience "highs and lows" from fluctuations in glucose levels. When glucose goes low for example, the brain is starved of this very essential element for its proper functioning and can cause the person having the hypoglycemic episode to act strangely and present with spells of bizarre behaviors. Severe hypoglycemia can actually cause a person to hallucinate and to experience short term memory loss.

People with wide swings in glucose have also been known to pass out and if not treated, they can also risk diabetic coma. Hypoglycemia also causes adrenaline surges, which is the body's way of trying to compensate for low glucose, which can produce obvious anxiety symptoms. Adversely, hyperglycemic episodes (too much glucose in the blood) can make a person feel sleepy - both being the opposite of what you would think should happen. These factors might cause the one observing them to think they are experiencing a mental or emotional disorder.

Medical blood testing is typically not that expensive, so should be ordered, so that if a medical condition does exist, it can be treated and the resulting effect will be improvement of all symptoms, including the emotional ones.

If a patient needs the addition of medications to help with emotional symptoms, this can also be considered between the Doctor and patient, at the appropriate time during the treatment process.

One disease for example, that commonly causes anxiety and depression as part of its symptoms is thyroid disease as I mention above that affected me and that can result in hyperthyroidism (over-active thyroid) in some patients and hypothyroidism (under-active thyroid) in others. Of course there are many other diseases that cause emotional symptoms as well but the two I have so far mentioned, are prime examples.

Dr. Richard Hall MD and a professor of psychiatry, who has been involved in research studies at major medical universities such as John Hopkins University, has found in his studies, a direct relationship between anxiety and endocrine disorders. It was found in one study he directed, that in patients with "Hashimoto's thyroiditis/disease" (common autoimmune cause of hypothyroidism), anxiety was a common, initial and prominent symptom at the time patients were diagnosed.

There are also studies that have been published on the "PubMed" (U.S. National Institutes of Health) website, which is provided by the National Library of Medicine, that state that anxiety symptoms and anxiety disorders are directly associated with Hashimoto's disease. This is in addition to depression, has been known to be a symptom of thyroid diseases for many years.

I believe if a hypothyroid patient for example, is on adequate treatment/hormone replacement therapy but still needs the added help of an antidepressant, there is nothing at all wrong with this!

Identifying and Treating Mental and Emotional Disorders

Having said this, let me now point out problems I see with Doctors who do not first give thyroid hormone replacement time to work, before adding an antidepressant to a patient's treatment. Certainly thyroid hormone therapy and any other hormone therapy, has the potential to relieve symptoms greatly. I'll say in my own case for example, that the emotional symptoms were the ones helped the most and the first to resolve when I was treated for thyroid disease and this alone was a great accomplishment for me.

Help with prescribed medication for anxiety, is nothing to be ashamed of or afraid of either, if it is needed while your thyroid treatment is being optimized, which can actually take several months. Dose adjustments are often needed, for as much as a year after beginning an initial dose. Some medical sources imply that thyroid hormone replacement therapy for hypothyroid conditions, takes only 4 to 6 weeks to do its job properly but this simply is not true with a large percent of patients, who may need several dosage adjustments, before they reach their optimal treatment level.

What was not good in my case and in the case of many other fellow thyroid patients I have corresponded with whom have experienced the same scenario as I, is the "snap diagnosed" emotional only problems that can occur. In my case the thyroid disease was not blood-tested for until I demanded that the tests be ordered. Because of this, my fatigue, joint pain, dry skin, etc...., did not improve on the antidepressant alone but actually worsened.

This combination of worsening hypothyroidism and the side effects of the SSRI-antidepressant I was prescribed resulted in my weaning off the drug very slowly.

Identifying and Treating Mental and Emotional Disorders

In the mean time, blood tests I demanded and had blood drawn for, just prior to starting the mood drugs, clearly revealed thyroid disease, including hypothyroidism and highly elevated thyroid antibody levels (thyroid autoimmunity).

The problem I saw in my original GP pushing constantly for me to resume the antidepressant, along with my thyroid hormone medication, was that there was the potential for me to confuse the SSRI side-effects, with unrelieved thyroid disease symptoms. The side-effects after all, include some that are identical to thyroid disease; "fatigue, tremor, nervousness, lightheadedness etc..."

In my opinion, thyroid disease symptoms, including depression/anxiety, should be monitored with hormone treatment, to see how well they improve and if they do not begin to improve significantly after a few weeks on the replacement therapy, an SSRI and other medications, such as those for muscle/joint aches etc..., can then be added. I believe if anxiety and/or depression is thyroid disease related, obviously hormone replacement has an even greater potential to improve it, than an antidepressant does. This is not to say that a combination of these treatments might not be needed at some point.

Another problem is "withdrawal" from SSRI drugs and other medications designed to treat emotional disorders. Patients, who have been on an antidepressant for months or years, will experience a worsening of their emotional symptoms, plus other withdrawal symptoms, when weaning off of an antidepressant and is why it must be done very slowly under doctor supervision. They may mistakenly believe this indicates that the emotional symptoms are becoming more severe without the SSRI or other drug.

In reality, this is a common reaction (worsening emotions and other withdrawal side-effects) when tapering off of one.

If a patient, with Doctor-supervision decides to taper off of an antidepressant, it must be done very slowly, with withdrawal symptoms monitored closely because some patients actually have been known to become suicidal during withdrawal, while others don't have as difficult a time.

If a medical disorder patient does not have a problem with the possibility of needing antidepressants as lifelong treatment and they do indeed need the drug for emotional symptoms (and many do), they should make the decision to remain on them for as long as is necessary. If at some point they want to wean off of the drug, it should be done slowly and very cautiously and never without Doctor Supervision.

While antidepressant medications are very helpful and necessary under the right conditions, consideration should also be given to the possibility of underlying medical causes of emotional symptoms that must also be diagnosed and treated, with adequate time for disease-treatment to resolve symptoms as stated earlier.

When patients who are prescribed antidepressants do not adjust well to them, trials of other types of psychotropic drugs should be considered or types that are used only as-needed. Doctors can also suggest therapies or refer the patient for specific therapy treatments including Cognitive Behavioral Therapy.

CHAPTER TEN:

More Patent-Education and Doctor-Communication about SSRI Antidepressants

In this chapter, I wish to express some further opinions about SSRI antidepressants in-general, that come from my years of correspondence with both doctors and patients on the subject and from several years of extensive online search on the subject.

What an amazing subject SSRI antidepressants are, with so many controversies and conflicting opinions out there about them! It is an interesting subject however and one I've searched and researched many times since the year 2003. My searching was also prompted by the fact that I had five Doctors in succession try to prescribe SSRI antidepressants to me, early into my own treatment for hypothyroidism because of my experiencing some unresolved symptoms after treatment with thyroid hormone replacement therapy.

These Doctors felt that the thyroid hormone therapy I was taking for hypothyroidism was always highly successful in all patients and that my unresolved symptoms must have been psychosomatic or simply emotional ones. Once I received the correct dose of thyroid medication however, the symptoms they claimed were psychosomatic resolved significantly over time. In the mean time, I researched about SSRI drugs because of my experience with so many doctors wanting to prescribe them. I was also hearing from many other fellow-patients who were continually being suggested or prescribed SSRI drugs by their Doctors, I simply had to know more about why they were being prescribed so commonly.

44

Let me say again, that I sincerely believe these drugs do have a purpose and that there are people who greatly benefit from them. At times they have actually prevented suicides, as some patients will attest. On the other side of the coin however, is the fact that Doctors fall into the habit of prescribing these type drugs at every turn so-to-speak because they have convinced of their widespread compatibility by the pharmaceutical companies who manufacture them.

Some Doctors fail to recognize the fact that there are those people the drugs might not be compatible with, who experience adverse reactions to them if they are not needed or they are experiencing a medical condition needing attention. Some of these type reactions have included suicidal tendencies. While this is not common, the FDA now requires mention of this possibility of the labels of these drugs. I feel with the possibility of severe side effects, patients or the parents of patients (if they are minors) that are prescribed SSRI antidepressants should be thoroughly monitored while adjusting to the drugs and sufficiently educated about them.

I feel they should also have a hotline to their Doctors when starting these drugs and told to report the first signs of threatening side effects. Doctors should also be willing to carefully switch patients to a different type medication if one has adverse effects, rather than telling the patient that the side effects are imagined or a sign that their emotions were on the verge of getting worse but caught just in time and that they were simply needing a dose increase of the SSRI drug.

Doctors don't always thoroughly inform patients about these possible adverse or negative possibilities.

They are routinely briefed by the pharmaceutical companies who insist that the drugs can be mass prescribed with very little chance of any adverse effects in the population of those they are administered to.

There are caring, compassionate people who work for and head the companies who manufacture psychotropic drugs but a main driving force behind them is marketing and sales (market shares). Again, this does not take away from the fact that the drugs are greatly beneficial to many people they are prescribed to but prescribing abuse is also a reality with some of these types of drugs. There is balance needed between manufacturers and doctors because one represents marketing, while the other represents a calling to heal and preserve the lives and best health-interests of the end-recipient patients.

The reason the FDA has had to step in and require stricter measures in regard to the warnings on labels of SSRI drugs, is because severe, adverse reactions were occurring in some patients taking them and the manufacturers of the drugs did not want a great deal of press in regard to this fact. Some even fought legally to keep from having to add warnings about adverse reactions on the prescribed drugs labels.

There are actually several areas of concern, including those previously mentioned, in regard to SSRI antidepressants that simply require more Doctor and patient education and communication. Patients in need of a trial of one of these drugs may not have the energy to read a long patient print-out that is offered with the medication so they need their Doctor to brief them on all areas of concern in regard to the drugs. One example in this area is the fact that some SSRI drugs and other types of antidepressants require patients who take them to abstain from alcohol but is a warning their Doctors may fail to inform them about.

Identifying and Treating Mental and Emotional Disorders

In regard to SSRI drugs lowering thyroid hormones in the body, in some people who take them, I read about this possibility years ago, in articles published on reputable medical research websites after I was diagnosed with thyroid disease. The fact that some of these drugs can indeed do this was included in medical research articles and not just the opinion of non-medical people. In people who take thyroid hormone replacement, this may result in a need to raise their hormone medication dose.

In people who aren't clinically hypothyroid however, taking an SSRI long term, might present the need for them to have their thyroid hormone levels tested every few months, to see if they are a patient whose levels are significantly affected by the drug. Most patient's, own bodies will adjust their thyroid hormone levels if the drug lowers them over time but this might not be true in all cases, especially in elderly patients. Here again, is a need for Doctor and patient education about the possible reactions caused by these drugs.

If I were to sum up my opinion on the subject of prescribed psychotropic drugs, I would say that I believe many people are greatly helped by them but I also believe some people have adverse reactions to them. I believe because of this, Doctors need to brief patients better about these type facts that I have addressed, rather than assuming they are safe and effective for all patients, in all cases.

Certainly the only way to know if a patient will benefit who is legitimately determined to be in need of a psychotropic drug, is to place them on a trial of one. They are powerful drugs however and in my opinion, it is extremely important that Doctors and patients become better educated about them.

They should communicate adequately in regard to them as treatment is being administered.

Are There Effective Natural Anxiety Treatments?

Yes, there are natural supplements, including some herbals that are reported to be helpful to some anxiety patients by calming the nervous system. I mention some of these in anxiety-subject articles I have written. I do however believe that a person should approve any supplement through their doctor. The U.S. National Institutes of Health lists natural supplements on one of their sites, explaining their uses and what they have learned about them through their research. It is a reputable source for the evaluation of natural supplements in my opinion.

Following are two anxiety herbals they give information on and you can find others using their alphabetized categories at the top of these pages.

"Valerian" -- Quote: "Several studies of valerian have reported benefits in reducing non-specific anxiety symptoms."

"Kava"-- Quote: "Human studies have found at least moderate benefit of kava in the treatment of anxiety, and early evidence suggests that kava may be as effective as benzodiazepine drugs such as diazepam (Valium®)."

<u>CHAPTER ELEVEN:</u>

Stress Management to Aid Treatments for Mind and Emotions

Stress can continually be a major problem in a person's life especially in these days of living in this crazy, hectic, fast-paced world. Stress can be brought on and aggravated by many things both major and minor including the following.

- work
- personal life problems
- financial issues
- relationships
- school
- children
- health problems

Many times stress builds from an overload of all these things combined. Some people even become stressed over the little things such as traffic, a long line at the grocery store, house chores and upcoming events or even because a waiter treated them badly at a restaurant. These are just a few examples of common stressors and there are many things that cause stress in people's lives that can accumulate and become harmful over time.

There are many stress-relievers available for practice to help us deal with the "stressors" of daily life. Yoga and meditation are very popular ways that can help us experience some relief from the stressors of a hectic life. Exercise in general is also a great way to deal with excessive stress.

Having an occasional quiet time can also provide some stress reduction, by removing ourselves from everything and everyone for a few minutes each day, for some quiet, alone time. This can help us to calm-down and place us back into focus. Deep breathing exercises are another good way to relieve stress, by taking, slow, long, deep breaths, inflating your diaphragm (stomach), rather than your chest.

Some people suffer stress that is severe enough that they need the help of a therapist to deal with it. This can actually be a good idea if one is suffering stress severe enough that they begin to lose the ability to handle it well on their own or it is causing them emotional problems. Hobbies and leisure activities that are enjoyed can also be stress relievers. Activities involving art projects, such as painting, drawing, building things, scrap-booking, and gardening are a few simple ways to get one's mind off of all the stressors being experienced and to enjoy some leisure time.

The consequences of not mastering or at least improving the skill of stress management may include health problems, depression, and lack of sleep to name a few. Stress can contribute-to or can even be a cause of these health issues that can be potentially harmful if it is not brought under reasonable control. Other health problems caused-by or contributed-to by stress may also include the following.

• muscle tension
• increased heart rate
• headaches
• increased blood pressure (hypertension)
• increased risk for heart attack and stroke
• more vulnerability to colds and viruses
• increase the risk for developing certain types of diseases

Stress can also take away much the happiness in life and cause symptoms of anxiety and an increased susceptibility to depression. For these reasons it is very important to work on skills for mastering stress.

Other ways for gaining stress management would include identifying all of the things that stress you out and to begin working on improving these areas. A simple method for helping to identify stressors is to write them down in a notebook each time you find yourself getting stressed about something. This will help you identify those stressors, so that you can begin to work on ways to better deal with and reduce them and to possibly eliminate them. Also, try working on ways to stop any negative thought patterns that contribute to stress as soon as they begin coming into your mind. Try to think positively no matter what situation may arise because it is very likely that your concerns are not as serious as you have allowed yourself to think or believe they are.

You have to develop a practice of controlling your negative responses to stressful thoughts and learn to better cope with them. Also try to remove yourself from any situations that cause added stress for you, whether it is certain job situations or even a relationship that causes you undue stress. If you can identify anything that is negatively affecting your daily life, it is important to remove yourself from those things if at all possible, since they will only serve to make life more difficult and complicated than it should reasonably have to be.

Most people can benefit in many ways from mastering these skills for reducing stress which can lend toward a much happier and healthier life. The benefits of better health that can result are not only physical but also mental and emotional.

Identifying and Treating Mental and Emotional Disorders

Mastering these skills can also help you to benefit more from life itself and help you to experience more enjoyment as well.

Hopefully more people will begin to realize that chronic stress is a continually growing problem in our society and may actually cause negative and violent behaviors in some people. We all must begin working more on skills and methods for coping because stress can easily spiral out of control if we do not do everything we can to control it instead of allowing it to control us.

Are There Self-Help Therapies for Anxiety Disorder?

One of the most effective therapies which can also be self-administered in addition to getting it from a mental health professional is "Cognitive Behavioral Therapy" (CBT) as discussed in previous chapters. The method helps one to react differently to emotions that tend to become imbalanced if reactions to them are not changed. It is a therapy that takes some time and practice but has a high treatment success rate. It also helps you to not fear the symptoms of strong emotion and to change your behavior in response to them, which over times diminishes their effects in hindering your ability to carry on normal life and activities. You also start to recognize these emotions as being natural in their proper context, so that you have less fear and dread of them.

In my opinion, CBT methods are the best in learning to cope-with and possibly completely overcome anxiety and depression. It worked for me tremendously well when I suffered severe anxiety symptoms and panic attacks from the onset of thyroid disease and other co morbid health disorders I experienced.

One source you might search-out if you are looking for anxiety self-help resources, is the "National Association of Cognitive-Behavioral Therapists", which also gives updates on CBT self-help programs they recommend, as they become available. A general search on CBT will also yield you lots of helpful information.

People experiencing the emotional or mental disorders discussed in the preceding chapters and the family, friends and associates of these patients, should be aware of how commonly these disorders co-exist but should also learn about the major features that help distinguish between them for more targeted treatments.

(END)